Ways to lead a healthy life: are we ready?

Preface

One of the most important questions of our life and we need to ask this question to ourselves frequently which is nothing but – am I healthy?

People are running around the busy work schedule ignoring the importance of health forcing them to take a break around the age of 45 to 50 and think seriously about their health. If the break is shorter they are lucky enough to continue the way they want. If the break is longer, it affects the earning power, mobility, dependence on others, affecting short and long term plans of our life and in the worst case it leads to the ultimate.

Number of articles, tips and books are written in this topic still we are not able to achieve the desired level of healthy life. In the present scenario most of the health related issues arise either due to stress, lack of awareness, laziness, ignorance, food habit, environment, procrastination and heredity.

When we list down the reasons and causes for the health issues, we will be able to find most of the reasons are controllable and possible with the change in attitude and life style.

Different systems of treatment such as Allopathic, Ayurvedic, Unony, Homeopathy available to overcome the health issues but prevention is always better than cure and we should educate ourselves and our children. The book throws light on the various health issues which are controllable and help the readers to lead a healthy life.

Author wishes the readers a Happy and Healthy life
Health Researcher

Contents

According to World Health Organization (WHO) the average life expectancy in the year 1955 was 48 years and it is increased to 65 years in 1995. It is estimated to be 73 years in 2025. The improvement was made possible through various measures taken at the global and country level in the health care sector.

The global population was 2.8 billion in 1955 and it is estimated to be 8 billion in 2025. Currently 3.1 billion adults are in the age group 20-64. Old population vs. young population ratio will be 31/100 during 2025 which was 16/100. This will pose a challenge in terms of maintaining healthy life at the old age

According to World health organization global estimates (2016) figures the leading cause of mortality are communicable, maternal, perinatal and nutritional conditions accounts for 20.1%, non-communicable disease account for 71.3% and injuries account for 8.6%.

Out of the non-communicable disease cardiovascular disease accounts for 31.4% and digestive disease accounts for 4.5% summing up to 1/3 of the total percentage. The top 20 disease shows that Ischemic heart disease (10.6%), Stroke (10.2%) and Diabetes mellitus (2.8%) which accounts for 1/ 4th of the total percentage.

Though these mortality indicators are the effect of different factors we cannot ignore the life style factor. For instance the percentage of cardiovascular disease related mortality at the age group 30-60 accounts for 18% and 10% in Male and females respectively.

Cardiovascular disease mortality

Age Group	Male	Female
0-28 days	0.01%	0.01%
1-59 months	0.19%	0.17%
5-14 years	0.13%	0.13%
15-29 years	1.15%	0.79%
30-49 years	7.56%	4.22%
50-59 years	12.15%	6.98%
60-69 years	22.30%	16.17%
70+ years	56.52%	71.53%

There is also a positive correlation seen between life style related causes and the mortality i.e. the non-communicable disease related mortality is more in high and upper income group according to World Health Statistics 2019 report.

References

1. https://www.who.int/whr/1998/media_centre/50facts/en/
2. https://www.who.int/healthinfo/global_burden_disease/estimates/en/
3. https://apps.who.int/iris/bitstream/handle/10665/324835/9789241565707-eng.pdf?ua=1

Life style has a huge impact on healthy life. Healthy life style component includes right diet, adequate physical activity, yoga, right habits and regular health checkup.

Component of Healthy life style

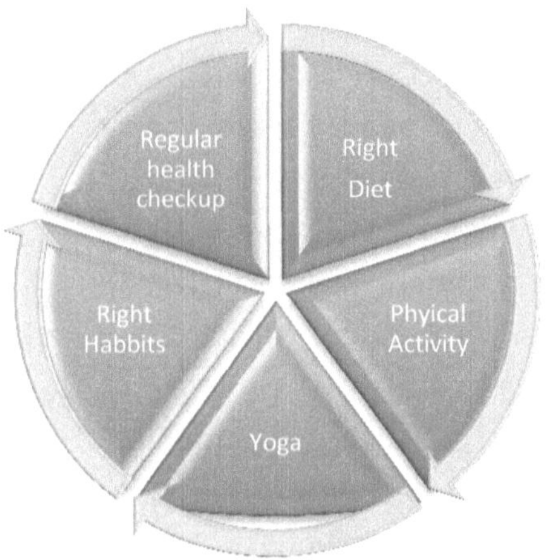

The Nurses' Health Study (NHS) and the Health Professionals Follow-up Study conducted provided valuable insights on effect of habits on the health. The study found people with healthy life style had longer and comfortable life and not affected by the non-communicable disease like cardiovascular disease.

There are numerous studies conducted on the effect of life style on the health.

References

1. http://www.euro.who.int/en/media-centre/sections/fact-sheets/2014/09/food-and-nutrition
2. Hu, F. B., & Willett, W. C. (2001). Diet and coronary heart disease: findings from the Nurses' Health Study and Health Professionals' Follow-up Study. The journal of nutrition, health & aging, 5(3), 132-138.
3. Chiuve, S. E., Rexrode, K. M., Spiegelman, D., Logroscino, G., Manson, J. E., & Rimm, E. B. (2008). Primary prevention of stroke by healthy lifestyle. Circulation, 118(9), 947.
4. King, D. E., Mainous III, A. G., & Geesey, M. E. (2007). Turning back the clock: adopting a healthy lifestyle in middle age. The American journal of medicine, 120(7), 598-603.
5. Visser, M., Wijnhoven, H. A., Comijs, H. C., Thomése, F. G., Twisk, J. W., & Deeg, D. J. (2019). A healthy lifestyle in old age and prospective change in four domains of functioning. Journal of aging and health, 31(7), 1297-1314.

Right diet is needed to lead a healthy life. Human body needs the following important nutrients. Men require approximately 2400 calories a day and women require 2000 calories per day.

Carbohydrates

Carbohydrates provide required energy to the human body in the form glucose. The following food items contains significant amount of carbohydrates

Nuts	Grains	Fruits	Vegetables	Animal Products
Almond	Cereals	Apple	Potatoes	Milk
Peanut	Bread	Orange	Beans	Yogurt
Sunflower seeds	Rice	Pear	Asparagus	Chicken
	Pasta	Apricots	Broccoli	Meat
		Banana	Carrot	Beef
		Blueberries	Tomato	Egg
		Raspberries	Spinach	Pork
		Cantaloupe		
		Figs		
		Plums		
		Kiwi		
		Pineapple		
		Papaya		
		Prunes		
		Raisins		
		watermelon		

Proteins

Proteins are important component in our cells growth and play a vital role in producing hormones and enzymes. The following food items contains significant amount of proteins

Nuts	Grains	Fruits	Vegetables	Animal Products
Peanut	Wheat	Guava	Soya beans	Egg
Flax seeds	Oatmeal	Avocados	Lentils	Fish
Pumpkin seeds		Apricots	Beans	Milk
Sunflower seeds		Kiwi	Peas	Yogurt
Almond		Cantaloupe	Spinach	Cheese
Walnuts		Bananas	Tofu	Meat

Vitamins

Vitamins are essential for the body to function normally. Body requires different types of Vitamins such Vitamin A, B, C, D, E and K. Each vitamin plays different role in the functioning of the human body such as

- Maintaining the bone density
- Healthy nervous system
- Growth of hormones,
- Healthy Vision
- Healthy skin
- Enabling blood clotting
- Blood production

Vitamin A	Vitamin B	Vitamin C	Vitamin D	Vitamin E	Vitamin K
Apricot	Peanut	Orange	Egg	Almond	Green leafy Vegetables
Cantaloupe	Egg	Mango	Fish	Avocado	Spinach
Avocado	Fish	Guava	Soya beans	Sunflower seeds	Asparagus
Milk	Milk	Banana	Mushrooms	Spinach	
Cheese	Brown rice	Kiwi	Milk	Asparagus	
Broccoli	Wheat	Strawberries			
Peas	Oatmeal	Pineapple			
Spinach	Raspberries	Apricot			
Sweet Potato	Lychee	Apple			
Cabbage	Pineapple	Lemon			
Carrot	Avocado	Blackberry			
Tomato	Corn	Papaya			
	Broccoli	Broccoli			
	Cabbage	Tomato			

Minerals

Minerals ensure the tissues and fluids in the body works properly. The following minerals such as Calcium, Iron, Iodine, Potassium, Zinc and Sodium keep the body healthier.

Calcium	iron	Folic Acid	Iodine	Potassium	Sodium
Almond	Soybeans	Broccoli	Egg	Orange	Salt
Orange	Spinach	Corn	Fish	Potatoes	
Fish	lentils	Green leafy Vegetables	Milk	Lemon	
Milk	Beans	Beans	Yogurt	Banana	
Yogurt	Green leafy Vegetables	Sunflower seeds	Cereals	Cantaloupe	
Green leafy Vegetables	Mushroom	Egg		Beet greens	
Soy milk	Beef	Fish		Prunes	
Broccoli	Egg				
Spinach	Chicken				
	Fish				
	Peanut				
	Dates				
	Apricot				
	Peaches				
	Prunes				

Fiber

Fiber is essential for the digestive system to function properly. It helps to reduce constipation. Fiber helps the body to absorb the nutrients present in the food items.

Nuts	Grains	Fruits	Vegetables
Almond	Brown rice	Prunes	Peas
Peanut	Wheat	Avocado	Beans
Walnut	Oatmeal	Blueberries	Artichoke
Lentils	Barley	Pear	Pumpkin
Pistachios		Raspberries	

Water

Water helps the body to absorb other nutrient and improve the functioning of digestive systems and carries oxygen to cells.

Fats

Fats provide the required energy for the body and it also helps the body to store fat soluble Vitamins A and D. Excessive fat will result in excess body weight as the body fails to burn the calories generated by the fat.

Daily intake components

Your diet should contain the combination fruits, vegetables, grains, mean and dairy group items. The possible combination of components of your daily intake is given in the chart below:

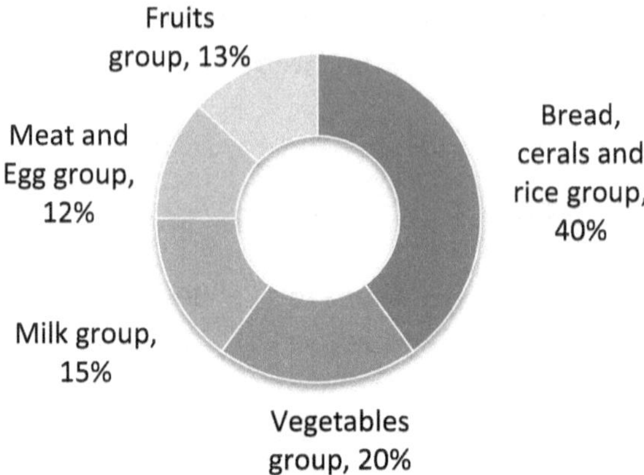

Components of daily intake for non vegans
Fruits group, 13%
Meat and Egg group, 12%
Milk group, 15%
Vegetables group, 20%
Bread, cerals and rice group, 40%

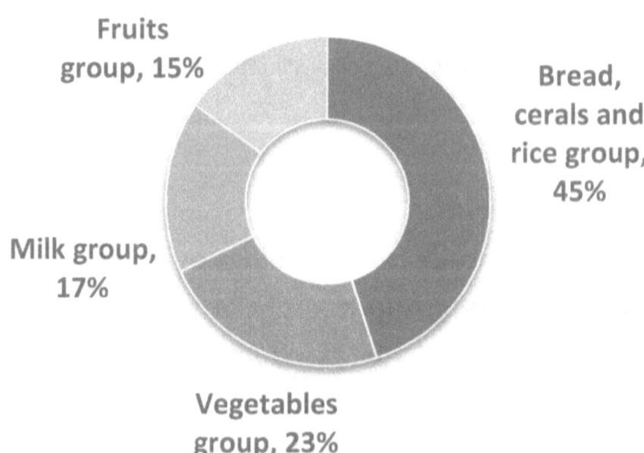

Components of daily intake for vegans
Fruits group, 15%
Milk group, 17%
Vegetables group, 23%
Bread, cerals and rice group, 45%

Percentage of Fat, Protein and Carbohydrates

The possible percentage of Fat, Protein and Carbohydrates are given in the below chart. It includes almost 50% carbohydrates which is needed for providing energy

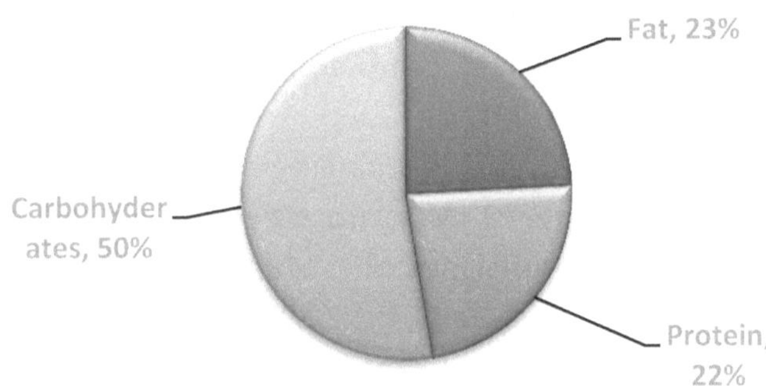

Food to avoid

The following food items needs to be avoided

- Saturated fat
- Trans fatty acid
- Consumption of excessive sugar (maximum 10% of total energy) salt (maximum 5g per day)
- Sweetened beverages
- Processed meats

References

1. World Health Organization. (2004). Vitamin and mineral requirements in human nutrition. World Health Organization.
2. Tolonen, M. (1990). Vitamins and minerals in health and nutrition. Elsevier.
3. Melini, V., & Melini, F. (2019). Gluten-free diet: gaps and needs for a healthier diet. Nutrients, 11(1), 170.
4. Incze, M. (2019). Vitamins and Nutritional Supplements: What Do I Need to Know?. JAMA internal medicine, 179(3), 460-460.
5. Ramya, V., & Patel, P. (2019). Health benefits of vegetables. IJCS, 7(2), 82-87.
6. Marino, M. (2019). HEALTHY NATURAL DIET: the hnd method. Dr. Mariano Marino.
7. Sammugam, L., & Pasupuleti, V. R. (2019). Balanced diets in food systems: emerging trends and challenges for human health. Critical reviews in food science and nutrition, 59(17), 2746-2759.
8. Webb, G. P. (2019). Nutrition: maintaining and improving health. CRC Press.
9. Thiele, S., Mensink, G. B., & Beitz, R. (2004). Determinants of diet quality. Public health nutrition, 7(1), 29-37.

Any one of the below mentioned physical activities are essential to lead a healthy life style. Physical activities will be useful based on the three characteristics its intensity, duration of the activity and frequency of the activity.

- Walking
- Jogging
- Exercise
- Cycling
- Swimming

Walking

In terms of the intensity, walking is the least out of the above 5 physical activity. Walking is one of the physical activities which can be continued longer period in one's life due to easy adoption, no formal training is required and irrespective of the fitness level. Brisk walking for 30 minutes per day is suggested. We need to walk whenever there is an opportunity exists like walking to the nearest bus stop, stores, stair case when possible. Walking has reduced risk of injuries when compared to running. Suitable time for walking will be either early morning or evening time, places near the park or beach side. It is preferred to use a sports shoe when walking. Time spent on walking is correlated with cardiovascular disease incidence. Walking in results in the following benefits

- Increases blood circulation and heart rate
- Burns fat
- Strengthen legs and improves balance

Barriers in walking

Even though walking is simplest form of physical activity there are also barriers in walking

- Lack of time – perceived or real
- Availability of Suitable space or location
- Weather condition

We can overcome the barriers by starting with walking of very small duration i.e. instead of recommended 30 min per day we can start with 5 minutes daily and increase gradually.

Jogging/Running

Jogging/Running is more intense than walking and burns calories more than walking. It has the same benefit in terms of keeping healthy heart and life style. The following are the extra barriers of running apart from the barriers of walking

- Not suitable for all ages and depends on the fitness level
- May result in wear and tear of muscle tissues and strains

Exercise

Physical exercise is more intense than walking and running and burns more calories than walking and running. Specific exercise is also helps to keep specific body parts stronger and is essential for sports persons. Exercises are normally planned and carried out in structured manner. The following are benefits of regular exercise

- Improve the health of heart function
- Reduce the risk of hypertension and diabetes
- Reduce depression and anxiety
- Better sleep
- Strengthening bones

There are different types of exercises to increase heart rate, strengthen the bones, muscles and increase flexibility.

Aerobic exercise

Aerobic exercise which includes running and jogging also which helps us to keep healthy heart, reduce blood sugar level and blood pressure.

Strengthening

Strengthening exercise include lifting of weights, pushing arms in opposite direction. It helps to strengthen our muscles and improve bone strength.

Balance

Balance exercise includes standing one leg and lift knee of one leg. Balancing exercise helps us from falling mainly at the older age.

Stretching

Stretching exercise helps us to make our body parts more flexible. It helps us to reduce cramps in the muscles and improves free motion of body parts.

Exercise also has the same barriers as running and important fact that exercise needs to be started only the advice of doctor.

Swimming

Swimming is more rigorous in terms of intensity and it is also involves all the parts of our body and helps to keep our body fit and healthy. One important thing in swimming we need proper training before we start the activity.

The following needs to be considered before starting the activity

- Choice place
- Clean water or clean swimming pool
- Proper swimming wear
- Safety measures

Cycling

Cycling is also more rigorous in terms of intensity and it also includes most of our body parts and helps our body fit and healthy. Cycling also requires proper training before starting the activity. Cycling is more prone to accidents and physical injuries are common and we need to be careful while selecting the roads or places for cycling activity.

The following needs to be considered before starting the activity

- Helmet and shoes
- Proper wear
- Follow traffic rules
- Quiet environment

Reference

1. https://www.health.harvard.edu/staying-healthy/walking-your-steps-to-healths
2. Hanson, S., & Jones, A. (2015). Is there evidence that walking groups have health benefits? A systematic review and meta-analysis. Br J Sports Med, 49(11), 710-715.
3. https://www.c3health.org/wp-content/uploads/2017/07/C3-report-on-walking-v-1-20120911.pdf
4. Caspersen, C. J., Powell, K. E., & Christenson, G. M. (1985). Physical activity, exercise, and physical fitness: definitions and distinctions for health-related research. Public health reports, 100(2), 126.
5. Fletcher, G. F., Balady, G., Blair, S. N., Blumenthal, J., Caspersen, C., Chaitman, B., ... & Pollock, M. L. (1996). Statement on exercise: benefits and recommendations for physical activity programs for all Americans: a statement for health professionals by the Committee on Exercise and Cardiac Rehabilitation of the Council on Clinical Cardiology, American Heart Association. Circulation, 94(4), 857-862.

Yoga is also a physical activity which is originated from India. Yoga Sutras text written by Sage Patanjali around 5th century BC is a guiding force for Yoga. It is little bit different from other physical activity as it also plays an important role in keeping the mind healthier apart from the body. Yoga is also a structured activity which needs to be carried out under the supervision of "Yoga Guru".

Different types of Yoga also called yoga poses/Asana helps us to keep the mind in good condition which results in reducing depression and anxiety, healthy heart, improved breathing, lower cholesterol level, blood sugar and blood pressure.

Different types of Yoga

There are different types of Yoga such as Hatha yoga which includes Pranayama and Asana. Other yoga types of yoga are Ashtanga, Bikram, Iyengar, Restorative and Kripalu Yoga.

Hatha Yoga

Hatha yoga is the general form of Yoga which includes breathing control and asana.

Pranayama

It is a yoga which is used to control the breath starts with inhalation, exhalation and retention of breath. It helps to reduce anxiety and depression, increases oxygen flow and improves the function of lungs. There are four forms of Pranayama are practiced

Basic – Inhale, fill, hold air in the lungs and release the air slowly. Repeat the process for desired number of times

Ujayi – It is same as basic except it creates sound through nose while breathing

Dirgha – During breathing process three parts of the body i.e. lung, chest and stomach are involved. One nostril will be open and other will be closed while inhaling. While exhaling the other nostril will be open and opened nostril will be closed.

Nodi Sodhana – The breathing process takes places through only one nostril at a time.

Meditation

Meditation helps to improve the mental health and concentration. There are different forms of meditation is available

Mindful – We need to sit in a place and centering our attention by focusing on our breath or few words which are confortable for us

Concentration – We concentrate on only one physical thing around us for a particular period of time.

Ashtanga

Ashtanga yoga is a series of postures which continuously flowing in specific defined sequence. It helps to make our body flexible and strengthen muscles. It is also called eight limbed yoga and it is also linked to spirituality.

Bikram

It is also called hot yoga as it is usually carried out in hot room temperature to make the environment similar in India. It includes carrying out different asana in different sequence.

Iyengar

Iyengar yoga was promoted by a Yoga Guru Iyengar involves carrying out specific sequence of Asana carried with help of wooden gadgets, belts and ropes.

Restorative Yoga

Restorative yoga is used to relax our body and mind and use blankets and neck pillows. Usual posture in this yoga is to lie down in the ground and focus on our breath to get mind relaxed.

Kripalu Yoga

Kripalu yoga involves holding postures for a longer period of time along with controlling breath and carrying out meditation.

All the above type of Yoga to be carried out under the supervision of a Yoga Guru

Reference

1. Hartranft, C. (2003). The Yoga-sutra of Patanjali: a new translation with commentary. Shambhala Publications.
2. Taneja, D. K. (2014). Yoga and health. Indian journal of community medicine: official publication of Indian Association of Preventive & Social Medicine, 39(2), 68.
3. Wiese, C., Keil, D., Rasmussen, A. S., & Olesen, R. (2019). Effects of yoga asana practice approach on types of benefits experienced. International journal of yoga, 12(3), 218.
4. Streeter, C. C., Jensen, J. E., Perlmutter, R. M., Cabral, H. J., Tian, H., Terhune, D. B., ... & Renshaw, P. F. (2007). Yoga Asana sessions increase brain GABA levels: a pilot study. The journal of alternative and complementary medicine, 13(4), 419-426.
5. Maehle, G. (2007). Ashtanga Yoga: Practice and Philosophy: A comprehensive description of the primary series of ashtanga Yoga, following the traditional vinyasa count, and an authentic explanation of the

Overweight

Right weight according to height will be an important factor in deciding our obesity status. To know the obesity status we can use the Body Mass Index which is calculated from the below given formula

Body Mass Index (BMI) = weight in kilograms / (height in meters)^2

If a person weighs 90 kg and his height is 1.8 meters then BMI is calculated as 27.7 and he will be in pre obesity status as per the below table

BMI	Nutritional status
Below 18.5	Underweight
18.5–24.9	Normal weight
25.0–29.9	Pre-obesity
30.0–34.9	Obesity class I
35.0–39.9	Obesity class II
Above 40 O	Obesity class III

Obesity may cause several diseases such as diabetes mellitus, cardio vascular and blood pressure.

Ways to overcome overweight

Obesity or overweight is a preventable condition or disease. To prevent or overcome overweight problem the following activities and food items are suggested

- Regular physical activity either walking, running and exercise to burn the excess calories
- Yoga – Ashtanga

- Food items
    - Use low fat food items
    - Avoid processed food times
    - Avoid sugar sweetened beverages
- Eat less and give gap between food intake
- Adequate Sleep

References

1. http://www.euro.who.int/en/health-topics/disease-prevention/nutrition/a-healthy-lifestyle/body-mass-index-bmi
2. North American Association for the Study of Obesity, National Heart, Lung, Blood Institute, & NHLBI Obesity Education Initiative. (2000). The practical guide: identification, evaluation, and treatment of overweight and obesity in adults. National Institutes of Health, National Heart, Lung, and Blood Institute, NHLBI Obesity Education Initiative, North American Association for the Study of Obesity.
3. Pi-Sunyer, F. X. (1993). Medical hazards of obesity. Annals of internal medicine, 119(7_Part_2), 655-660.

Diabetes Mellitus is a health condition wherein consistence high level of sugar presence in the blood. Normally the sugar which is released from the food items during digestion process enters the blood and will be absorbed by the cells with the help of hormone called insulin which is secreted from Pancreas. When the amount insulin secretion is reduced then sugar in the form of glucose released from the food items remains in the blood causing Diabetes Mellitus health condition.

There are two types of diabetes one is type 1 and another is type 2 diabetes. Type 1 diabetes is caused when immune system attacks our cells including pancreas which affects the secretion of insulin. Type 2 diabetes is caused when insufficient insulin is produced and due to which the blood sugar remains in the blood. Apart from these there is also a type called gestational diabetes which occurs only during pregnancy time in women.

Ways to prevent or keep diabetes under control

Diabetes mellitus (type 2 diabetes) is becoming a epidemic due to the changes in the life style, physical inactivity, influence of technology and change in the food habits and family history. To prevent or overcome the diabetes problem the following activities and food items are suggested

- Regular physical activity either walking, running and exercise to burn the excess calories
- Eat less and give gap between food intake to regulate the secretion of insulin

- Yoga – Ashtanga, Bikram, Iyengar
- Food items
    - Take food items rich in fiber content – Broccoli, Green leafy vegetables, beans
    - Fruits – Blueberries, raspberries
    - Avoid processed food times
    - Avoid sugar sweetened beverages

References

1. American Diabetes Association. (2013). Diagnosis and classification of diabetes mellitus. Diabetes care, 36(Supplement 1), S67-S74.
2. Kharroubi, A. T., & Darwish, H. M. (2015). Diabetes mellitus: The epidemic of the century. World journal of diabetes, 6(6), 850.
3. Eisenbarth, G. S. (1986). Type I diabetes mellitus. New England journal of medicine, 314(21), 1360-1368.
4. Buchanan, T. A., & Xiang, A. H. (2005). Gestational diabetes mellitus. The Journal of clinical investigation, 115(3), 485-491.
5. https://www.health.harvard.edu/a_to_z/diabetes-mellitus-overview-a-to-z

The high blood pressure or hypertension is linked to the size of arteries and the amount of blood the heart pumps into the arteries. If either heart pumps more blood and/or the arteries are narrower then it results in high blood pressure. High blood pressure condition will affect the heart's health severely. There are two types of hypertension one is primary and another secondary. The primary hypertension develops gradually and associated with aging while secondary hypertension is a result of some other diseases like kidney problem and sleep deprivation.

Ways to prevent or keep hypertension under control

- Yoga mainly meditation will help us to control the high blood pressure
- Likelihood of high blood pressure increases when we take high salt content in the food items
- We need to have the following high potassium rich food content to reduce the sodium
    - Banana
    - Orange
    - Apricot
    - Brocoli
    - Peas
    - Prunes
    - Dates

References

1. https://kcms-prod-mcorg.mayo.edu/diseases-conditions/high-blood-pressure/symptoms-causes/syc-20373410?p=1
2. National Collaborating Centre for Chronic Conditions (Great Britain). (2006). Hypertension: management in adults in primary care: pharmacological update. Royal College of Physicians.
3. Toledo, E., de A Carmona-Torre, F., Alonso, A., Puchau, B., Zulet, M. A., Martinez, J. A., & Martinez-Gonzalez, M. A. (2010). Hypothesis-oriented food patterns and incidence of hypertension: 6-year follow-up of the SUN (Seguimiento Universidad de Navarra) prospective cohort. Public health nutrition, 13(3), 338-349.
4. Karppanen, H., & Mervaala, E. (2006). Sodium intake and hypertension. Progress in cardiovascular diseases, 49(2), 59-75.

Heart or cardio vascular diseases includes different types of health condition such as artery related diseases, heart rythemic problems, heart failure or congenital defects.

The main reason of heart diseases is the accumulation of fats in the arteries resulting in atherosclerosis.

If the heart disease is It not treated it will result in heart attack, pain and stroke. The symptoms include chest pain, pain in left arm, shortness of breath, swelling in legs, fatigue and fever.

Ways to prevent or reduce the risk of heart diseases

- Regular Exercise
- Yoga – Asana and Meditation
- Low fatty food items
- Control type-2 diabetes and hypertension
- Controlled life style – non smoking and less alcohol intake
- Less salt
- Food items for healthy heart
  - High fiber
  - Oatmeal
  - Olive oil
  - Avocoda
  - Almond
  - Soybeans
  - Brocoli
  - Fish

References

1. Ulbricht, T. L. V., & Southgate, D. A. T. (1991). Coronary heart disease: seven dietary factors. The lancet, 338(8773), 985-992.
2. Castelli, W. P. (1984). Epidemiology of coronary heart disease: the Framingham study. The American journal of medicine, 76(2), 4-12.
3. Mackay, J., & Mensah, G. A. (2004). The atlas of heart disease and stroke. World Health Organization.
4. Vogel, R. A. (2019). Alcohol, heart disease, and mortality: a review. Reviews in cardiovascular medicine, 3(1), 7-13.
5. Powell, K. E., Thompson, P. D., Caspersen, C. J., & Kendrick, J. S. (1987). Physical activity and the incidence of coronary heart disease. Annual review of public health, 8(1), 253-287.
6. Stampfer, M. J., Hu, F. B., Manson, J. E., Rimm, E. B., & Willett, W. C. (2000). Primary prevention of coronary heart disease in women through diet and lifestyle. New England Journal of Medicine, 343(1), 16-22.

Some of the common problems or diseases related to eye are cataracts, glaucoma and retinal disorders and infection in the eyes.

Cataract is a result of clouding of the lens in the eyes which makes the vision blurred, creates double vision and increases the power of the glass which we wear. Development of cataract is also linked with aging.

Glaucoma is a result of optic nerve damages in the eyes.

Retinal disorders occur when the layers in the back of the eye are damaged. The layers are responsible for sensing and transmitting the images to the brain and also helping us to see the finer details.

Infection in the eye is caused by either bacteria or virus or allergies which make the eyes swell, itching and redness.

Ways to prevent or reduce risk of eyes diseases

The following precautions will helps us to prevent or reduce of risk of eye diseases

- Carry out Yoga and Meditation
- Give rest to your eyes
- Use sunglasses to protect from UV rays
- Eat food items such as
    - Fish which are high in omega-3 fatty acids
    - Green leafy vegetables
    - Control diabetes and hypertension
- Daily wash your eyes with clean water

References

1. Kertes, P. J., & Johnson, T. M. (Eds.). (2007). Evidence-based eye care. Lippincott Williams & Wilkins.

2. Olson, R. J., Mamalis, N., Werner, L., & Apple, D. J. (2003). Cataract treatment in the beginning of the 21st century. American journal of ophthalmology, 136(1), 146-154.

3. Smedley, G. T., Haffner, D., Niksch, B., Tu, H., & Burns, T. W. (2007). U.S. Patent No. 7,163,543. Washington, DC: U.S. Patent and Trademark Office.

4. Glaucoma treatment devicede - Juan Jr, E., Boyd, S., Deem, M. E., Gifford III, H. S., & Rosenman, D. (2014). U.S. Patent No. 8,721,656. Washington, DC: U.S. Patent and Trademark Office.

5. TNF inhibitors for the treatment of retinal disorders -Tobinick, E. L. (2002). U.S. Patent No. 6,379,666. Washington, DC: U.S. Patent and Trademark Office.

6. Friedman, N. J. (2010). Impact of dry eye disease and treatment on quality of life. Current opinion in ophthalmology, 21(4), 310-316.

The common ear related diseases are middle ear disease, Otosclerosis and hearing loss.

Middle ear disease is a result of bacterial or viral infection which affects the eardrums and builds fluids in the ear creating pain inside the ear.

Otosclerosis condition is wherein the bones in the ear grow abnormally.

Hearing loss is generally linked with aging when we fail to perceive the sound. The severity of the problem might be partial or total loss. The hearing process normally starts with the sound hitting the ear drums which vibrate and vibrations are amplified by the bones in the ear and transformed as nerve impulses transmitted to the brain.

Meniere's disease which is occurs when fluid accumulates in the inner ear causes hearing loss and ringing in the ear.

The vestibular system in the ear is responsible for the balance of the body which is affected when the ear get infected or injured.

Ways to prevent or reduce risk of eyes diseases

- Avoid the environment wherein the noise pollution is high or places where noises are loud
- Do not put any foreign objects into your ears.
- Vestibular exercises for balancing
- Intake low salt food

References

7. Kertes, P. J., & Johnson, T. M. (Eds.). (2007). Evidence-based eye care. Lippincott Williams & Wilkins.

8. Olson, R. J., Mamalis, N., Werner, L., & Apple, D. J. (2003). Cataract treatment in the beginning of the 21st century. American journal of ophthalmology, 136(1), 146-154.

9. Smedley, G. T., Haffner, D., Niksch, B., Tu, H., & Burns, T. W. (2007). U.S. Patent No. 7,163,543. Washington, DC: U.S. Patent and Trademark Office.

10. Glaucoma treatment devicede - Juan Jr, E., Boyd, S., Deem, M. E., Gifford III, H. S., & Rosenman, D. (2014). U.S. Patent No. 8,721,656. Washington, DC: U.S. Patent and Trademark Office.

11. TNF inhibitors for the treatment of retinal disorders -Tobinick, E. L. (2002). U.S. Patent No. 6,379,666. Washington, DC: U.S. Patent and Trademark Office.

12. Friedman, N. J. (2010). Impact of dry eye disease and treatment on quality of life. Current opinion in ophthalmology, 21(4), 310-316.

Cold is very common and seasonal especially occurs during winter affects the nasals. The cold condition is caused by infection in respiratory system near the nasals. It results in running nose, headache and sneezing.

Flu is an aggressive condition than cold as it is accompanied with high fever and body pain apart from other symptoms of cold. It is caused by influenza virus and mostly seasonal in nature. Type of Influenza virus changes every year and vaccines need to be produced based on the particular strains of the virus. People with heart or lung problems are at more risk than others.

Ways to prevent or control the impact of cold

Though cold lasts for a week the following measures will help prevent to control the impact of cold

- Take only hot water
- Take raw onion, ginger added green tea
- Keep your hands clean

Ways to prevent or control the impact of flu

Though flu looks similar to common cold but it can be dangerous event to the extreme condition. Hence it is advisable to take flu vaccination regularly and once you're diagnosed with flu take the following precautions.

- Take more fluid
- Take raw onion, ginger added green tea
- Do not smoke or take alcohol

References

1. Cold, S. C. The Flu. Nightime Relief. Acetaminophen, Doxylamine, Dextromethorphan, Alcohyl, 10(6).
2. Australia, H. (2019). Colds and flu–an overview.
3. Australia, H. (2019). Influenza A (flu).
4. Santos, J. C., & Matos, S. (2014). Analysing Twitter and web queries for flu trend prediction. Theoretical Biology and Medical Modelling, 11(1), S6.
5. Van Schoor, J. (2018). Combination cold and flu medication. Professional Nursing Today, 22(2), 4-6.
6. Van Schoor, J. (2018). Colds, flu and coughing: a review of over-the-counter cold and flu medicines. South African Family Practice, 60(3), 21-24.
7. Strauss, J. (2018). Complications from Flu–an unnecessary evil!. SA Pharmaceutical Journal, 85(3), 12-18.
8. Sanu, A., & Eccles, R. (2008). The effects of a hot drink on nasal airflow and symptoms of common cold and flu. Rhinology, 46(4), 271.

Sore throat is caused by viral or bacterial infection results in throat pain, difficulty in swallowing and affects the tonsils. Sore throat is also caused by allergies to medication.

Strep throat is a severe condition caused by bacteria called Streptococcus which is accompanied by fever, rashes, swollen tonsils.

Ways to prevent or control the impact of flu

Sore throat is normally present when we get affected by diseases like cold, flu and fever. If we control those diseases then pain from sore throat also we will be reduced. The following are the general precautions to avoid sore throat

- Keep your hands clean and use cleaned glasses
- Do not smoke or take alcohol
- Avoid things which are used by other people like public phones.

References

1. Del Mar, C., Glasziou, P. P., & Spinks, A. (2004). Antibiotics for sore throat. Cochrane database of systematic reviews, (2).
2. Ebell, M. H., Smith, M. A., Barry, H. C., Ives, K., & Carey, M. (2000). Does this patient have strep throat?. Jama, 284(22), 2912-2918.

Hypothyroid is caused by less amount thyroid produced by the thyroid gland in the body which is required in the body functioning such as regulating temperature, converting food and oxygen into energy. Hypothyroid is common in women than in men. It is associated with the symptoms of fatigue, intolerance to cold, skin problems, hair loss and weight gain.

Thyroid Stimulating Hormone (TSH) which is produced from the brain (pituitary gland) enables the thyroid gland to produce T4 and T3 cells and the same is released into the blood stream. Hypothyroid issues can be detected using Thyroid Stimulating Hormone (TSH) test and T4 test. If TSH is more then we need to do T4 test. If T4 is also low then hypothyroid problem is confirmed.

Ways to reduce the risk of hypothyroid

We can prevent or reduce the risk of developing hypothyroid issue by taking the following precautions

- Include iodized salt in your food preparation or intake as iodine is essential for the normal functioning of the Thyroid gland.
- Reduce the food items like soy, cabbage, cauliflower which may affect the Thyroid gland
- Food items such as egg, tuna Increase selenium levels in the body
- Food items which contains Vitamin Milk, and fish apart from getting exposure to sunlight

References

1. Cooper, D. S. (2001). Subclinical hypothyroidism. New England Journal of Medicine, 345(4), 260-265.
2. Hueston, W. J. (2001). Treatment of hypothyroidism. American family physician, 64(10), 1717-1724.
3. Gaitonde, D. Y., Rowley, K. D., & Sweeney, L. B. (2012). Hypothyroidism: an update. South African Family Practice, 54(5), 384-390.
4. Tonstad, S., Nathan, E., Oda, K., & Fraser, G. (2013). Vegan diets and hypothyroidism. Nutrients, 5(11), 4642-4652.
5. Hawkes, W. C., & Keim, N. L. (2003). Dietary selenium intake modulates thyroid hormone and energy metabolism in men. The Journal of nutrition, 133(11), 3443-3448.
6. Delange, F. (1994). The disorders induced by iodine deficiency. Thyroid, 4(1), 107-128.
7. Sharma, R., Bharti, S., & Kumar, K. H. (2014). Diet and thyroid-myths and facts. Journal of Medical Nutrition and Nutraceuticals, 3(2), 60.

Alzeimers disease is a health condition arises out of accumulation of proteins (tangles and plagques) which results in death of brain cells. It is one of the main cause of dementia and affects the thinking ability, ability to function independently.. Those affected by the disease will have the symptoms of not remembering the recent events and at the later stages results in the of improper use of words.

Ways to reduce the risk of Alzeimer disease

- Regular exercise
- Yoga and Meditation
- Good sleep
- Reading habit
- Involving in Social activities
- Aovid saturated fat food items
- Food times which reduces the risk of Alzeimer or dementia are
    - Beans
    - Green leafy vegetables
    - Nuts
    - Fish

References

1. Alzheimer's, A. (2015). 2015 Alzheimer's disease facts and figures. Alzheimer's & dementia: the journal of the Alzheimer's Association, 11(3), 332.

Anemia condition occurs when deficiency of hemoglobin and hematocrit found in the blood cells. The normal hemoglobin levels for men are 14 to 18 and 12 to 16 grams per deciliter. The normal level of hematocrit (% of red blood cells) is 40% to 50% in men and 35% to 45% in women.

Generally Anemia condition is caused by iron and vitamin deficiencies. Iron deficiency anemia is more common in women.

Ways to prevent or contol general anemia

Generally the anemic condition can be prevented using proper diet and vitamin supplements. Advanced forms of Anemia Aplastic, Sickle cell, Thalassemia anemic condition usually require blood transfusion.

- Take Iron, folic acid and vitamin B12 rich food times
  - Green leafy Vegetables
  - Dates
  - Beans
  - Egg
  - Nuts
  - Soy
  - Fish
  - Chicken
  - Milk
  - Yogurt
  - Cereals

References

1. Milman, N. (2011). Anemia—still a major health problem in many parts of the world!. Annals of hematology, 90(4), 369-377.
2. Yip, R. (2001). Iron deficiency and anemia. In Nutrition and health in developing countries (pp. 327-342). Humana Press, Totowa, NJ.
3. Kapur, D., Agarwal, K. N., & Agarwal, D. K. (2002). Nutritional anemia and its control. The Indian Journal of Pediatrics, 69(7), 607.
4. Weiss, G., & Goodnough, L. T. (2005). Anemia of chronic disease. New England Journal of Medicine, 352(10), 1011-1023.
5. Pauling, L., Itano, H. A., Singer, S. J., & Wells, I. C. (1949). Sickle cell anemia, a molecular disease. Science, 110(2865), 543-548.
6. Young, N. S., Scheinberg, P., & Calado, R. T. (2008). Aplastic anemia. Current opinion in hematology, 15(3), 162.
7. Dhaliwai, G., Cornett, P. A., & Tierney, L. M. (2004). Hemolytic anemia. American family physician, 69, 2599-2608.

Lungs play an important role in the breathing process and affected by diseases like Asthma, Tuberculosis and Bronchitis. Air pollution, Toxic work related environment also badly affects the functioning of the lungs.

Asthma is caused by the narrowing and swelling of air ways along with excessive secretion of mucus. It is accompanied with shortness of breath and wheezing.

Tuberculosis which affects the lungs is caused by bacteria which mostly transmitted from another person through droplets in the air.

Bronchitis is caused by inflammation in the bronchial tubes which helps the oxygen to pass in and out of lungs.

Lung related diseases are diagnosed using chest X ray, Pulmonary Function Test and Bronchoscopy.

Ways to prevent or reduce the impact of lung related diseases

- Yoga mainly pranayama plays an important role in controlling our breathing process including the lungs. Meditation also helps our lungs to function properly
- We need to use diaphragm muscles during the breathing process which differentiate the abdomen organ and the lungs
- We need to drink enough water and fluids which helps the lungs to perform better
- Avoid acid reflex
- Nonsmoking habit will help the lungs to function properly

- Avoid air pollution environment
- Use appropriate masks

References

1. National Heart, Lung, & Blood Institute. National Asthma Education Program. Expert Panel on the Management of Asthma. (1991). Guidelines for the diagnosis and management of asthma (No. 91). National Asthma Education Program, Office of Prevention, Education, and Control, National Heart, Lung, and Blood Institute, National Institutes of Health.
2. Flynn, J. L., & Chan, J. (2001). Immunology of tuberculosis. Annual review of immunology, 19(1), 93-129.
3. Cavanagh, D., & Naqi, S. A. (2003). Infectious bronchitis. Diseases of poultry, 11, 101-119.
4. Leuenberger, P., Künzli, N., Ackermann-Liebrich, U., Schindler, C., Bolognini, G., Bongard, J. P., ... & Keller, R. (1998). Swiss study on air pollution and lung diseases in adults (SAPALDIA). Schweizerische medizinische Wochenschrift, 128(5), 150-161.

Acid or Acid reflux is caused when acid in the stomach flows backward into the esophagus which differentiate stomach and Lungs. It creates heartburn sensation, upper abdominal pain and sore throat. It might result in continuous cough which may not be due cold or flu. It is measured by the term pH and it ranges from 0 to 14. If the pH value is 0 then it is totally acidic and if its 14 then alkaline will be more and will offset the acidity.

Ways to prevent or reduce the impact of acidity or acid reflux

The following precautions will help us to prevent or reduce the impact of acidity or acid reflux.

- Take food contents which are rich in alkaline which is essential to offset the effect of acidity
  - Yogurt
  - Egg White
  - Bananas
  - Oatmeal
  - Green leafy vegetables
- Avoid the following food items which are more acidic in nature
  - Fat related foods
  - Spicy food
  - Coffee
  - Tea
  - Tomato
  - Citrus fruits
  - Garlic

References

1. Nehra, D., Howell, P., Williams, C. P., Pye, J. K., & Beynon, J. (1999). Toxic bile acids in gastro-oesophageal reflux disease: influence of gastric acidity. Gut, 44(5), 598-602.
2. Fiorucci, S., Santucci, L., Chiucchiú, S., & Morelli, A. (1992). Gastric acidity and gastroesophageal reflux patterns in patients with esophagitis. Gastroenterology, 103(3), 855-861.
3. Boeckxstaens, G. E., & Smout, A. (2010). Systematic review: role of acid, weakly acidic and weakly alkaline reflux in gastro-oesophageal reflux disease. Alimentary pharmacology & therapeutics, 32(3), 334-343.
4. Feldman, M., Cryer, B., Sammer, D., Lee, E., & Spechler, S. J. (1999). Influence of H. pylori infection on meal-stimulated gastric acid secretion and gastroesophageal acid reflux. American Journal of Physiology-Gastrointestinal and Liver Physiology, 277(6), G1159-G1164.

Ulcers are caused by damages to the lining of stomach, small intestine or throat. Stomach ulcers are known as gastric ulcer, intestine ulcers are known as duodenal ulcers, digestive track ulcers are known as peptic ulcers and throat ulcers are known as esophagus ulcers. Ulcers cause pain, burning sensation and bloating. Ulcers are caused by Helicobacter Pylori bacteria.

Ulcers are diagnosed normally through blood test for H. Pylori bacteria and endoscopy.

Ways to prevent or reduce the impact of ulcer

- Take vitamin A and C rich foods
- Take the following fruits
    - Apple
    - Berries
    - Honey
    - Olive oil
    - Banana
- Meditation to relieve stress
- Avoid smoking and alcohal
- Good Sleep
- Avoid the following food items
    - Citrus fruits
    - Tomato
    - Coffee and Tea
    - Spicy food
    - Chocolate
    - Miik

References

1. Kurata, J. H., & Corboy, E. D. (1988). Current peptic ulcer time trends. An epidemiological profile. Journal of clinical gastroenterology, 10(3), 259-268.
2. Malfertheiner, P., Chan, F. K., & McColl, K. E. (2009). Peptic ulcer disease. The lancet, 374(9699), 1449-1461.
3. Kurata, J. H., & Haile, B. M. (1984). Epidemiology of peptic ulcer disease. Clinics in gastroenterology, 13(2), 289-307.
4. Rees, C. J., Pollack Jr, C. V., & Riese, V. G. (2019). Peptic Ulcer Disease. In *Differential Diagnosis of Cardiopulmonary Disease* (pp. 769-778). Springer, Cham.
5. Sverdén, E., Agréus, L., Dunn, J. M., & Lagergren, J. (2019). Peptic ulcer disease. Bmj, 367, l5495.
6. Mahima, M., Bhavesh, S., & Kumar, G. P. (2018). A REVIEW ON PEPTIC ULCER, ITS CAUSES AND TREATMENT.

Hernia is caused by weakening of abdominal wall and it causes intestine to come out of the abdomen and enters into parts below the abdomen. When it enters into the groin area then it is called inguinal hernia which usually occurs in men. There are two types of inguinal hernia one is direct hernia and another indirect inguinal hernia. Indirect hernia occurs when the inguinal canal fails to close before the birth.

Apart from inguinal hernia there are different types of hernia is present such as Femoral, Hiatal and Umbilical Hernia.

Femoral hernia is similar to inguinal hernia which occurs in women. In femoral hernia the intestine enters into the femoral blood vessel.

A hiatal hernia occurs when stomach pushes into diaphragm and to the chest region.

Umbilical hernia occurs when intestine bulges through umbilical card.

Normally hernia condition is cured through either open or laparoscopic surgeries

Ways to prevent or reduce the impact of hernia

- Avoid lifting of heavy weights
- Avoid constipation
- Avoid acidic food items
- Exercise which strength abdominal muscles
- Maintain correct BMI
- Include fiber rich food

References

1. Kingsnorth, A., & LeBlanc, K. (2003). Hernias: inguinal and incisional. The Lancet, 362(9395), 1561-1571.
2. Jenkins, J. T., & O'dwyer, P. J. (2008). Inguinal hernias. Bmj, 336(7638), 269-272.
3. Gilbert, A. I. (1992). Sutureless repair of inguinal hernia. The american journal of surgery, 163(3), 331-335.
4. Hachisuka, T. (2003). Femoral hernia repair. Surgical Clinics, 83(5), 1189-1205.
5. Wilson, L. J., Ma, W., & Hirschowitz, B. I. (1999). Association of obesity with hiatal hernia and esophagitis. The American journal of gastroenterology, 94(10), 2840.
6. Olmi, S., Scaini, A., Cesana, G. C., Erba, L., & Croce, E. (2007). Laparoscopic versus open incisional hernia repair. Surgical endoscopy, 21(4), 555-559.

Kidney is used to extract waste and excess water from blood and convert into urine. Kidney also helps us to remove acid from the cells and it also produces hormones which are essential to control blood pressure. When kidney is not functioning properly it leads to kidney failure, kidney infection and kidney stones.

Hemodialysis is a machine controlled process which extract the waste and excess water when the kidney not able to function completely.

Kidney stones are formed from the waste and become crystals and stays in the kidney. Kidney stones occur mainly due to less amount water intake.

Ways to prevent or reduce the impact of kidney diseases

- Reduce salt and potasium in your intake
- Drink enough water
- Do regular exercise
- Avoid smoking and alcohol
- We need to control diabetes and blood pressure
- The following food items to take
  - Fiber rich food items
  - Oatmeal
  - Fish
  - Soy protein
  - Yogurt
  - Egg

References

1. Levey, A. S., & Coresh, J. (2012). Chronic kidney disease. The lancet, 379(9811), 165-180.

2. Coe, F. L., Evan, A., & Worcester, E. (2005). Kidney stone disease. The Journal of clinical investigation, 115(10), 2598-2608.

3. Canaud, B., Kooman, J., Selby, N. M., Taal, M., Francis, S., Kopperschmidt, P., ... & Titze, J. (2019). Sodium and water handling during hemodialysis: new pathophysiologic insights and management approaches for improving outcomes in end-stage kidney disease. Kidney international, 95(2), 296-309.

4. Taylor, E. N., Fung, T. T., & Curhan, G. C. (2009). DASH-style diet associates with reduced risk for kidney stones. Journal of the American Society of Nephrology, 20(10), 2253-2259.

Varicose veins are twisted and enlarged veins found mainly in the legs. Persons who are working in an environment which required long hours of standing or more walking is affected by varicose vein disease. It causes itching, aching and pain in the legs.

Ways to prevent or reduce the impact of kidney diseases

- The normal treatment for varicose vein is to wear compression stockings
- Keep your legs in elevated position for some times.
- Change your siting and standing positions frequently
- Do regular exercise
- Take fiber rich food items

References

1. Callam, M. J. (1994). Epidemiology of varicose veins. British journal of surgery, 81(2), 167-173.
2. Houtermans-Auckel, J. P., van Rossum, E., Teijink, J. A. W., Dahlmans, A. A. H. R., Eussen, E. F. B., Nicolaï, S. P. A., & Welten, R. T. J. (2009). To wear or not to wear compression stockings after varicose vein stripping: a randomised controlled trial. European Journal of Vascular and Endovascular Surgery, 38(3), 387-391.